HATHA YOGA

MY BODY IS MY TEMPEL!

BESTSELLING AUTHOR

Shreyananda Natha

Cover & Graphic Design

Mattias Långström

Contact: oneofakindbooks@bhagwan.se

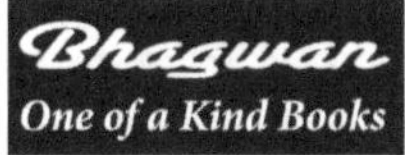

HATHA YOGA

MY BODY IS MY TEMPEL!

BESTSELLING AUTHOR

Shreyananda Natha

ISBN: 9789180207201

✳ ✳ ✳

Publisher: **BHAGWAN 2021**

Namasté

I want to thank the teachers and students I have had over the years and who have made my journey with yoga so interesting. Thank you for all the inspiration you have given me and for making this book possible. The yoga masters who no longer live among us – live on with every new person who immerses themselves in the yoga tradition: Sri Swami Sivananda, Sri Swami Satyananda, Sri Tirumalai Krishnamacharya, Sri Swami Vishnu-devananda, Sri K. Pattabhi Jois, Osho, Swami Nirdosha, Swami Omananda, Swami Janakanan-da, Ole Schmidt, Turiya, Maryam Abrishami and Sanna Kuittinen.

Everyone who has searched for answers to what they perceived through an activated ajna chakra. In yoga, they have learned the principles behind the universe, the collective consciousness, and the creative power, Kundalini Shakti. The duality behind everything, both what we see and what we do not see. Together we help to pass on the previous secret knowledge, about our gunas, nadis, and chakras, to anyone who wants to be a Siddha.

Aum Shri Durgayai Namaha – Shreyananda Natha.

THE AUTHOR

Shreyananda Natha is the author of over twelve titles on yoga. Among other things, he has written the most comprehensive books on yoga in Swedish, the Bestseller – ALL ABOUT YOGA and the study book – THE GREAT BOOK ABOUT YOGA. He is also a certified yoga and meditation teacher according to EYTF's international guidelines and has undergone a multi-year yoga teacher training under the leadership of Swami Omananda at Satyananda Ashram. Shreyananda Natha holds the highest initiation in the Tantric Natha Order. He travels frequently to Asia and India to improve himself, and to gain knowledge and inspiration. He has immersed himself in the tantric rituals and is known for his extensive knowledge of yoga, deep relaxation, and meditation

"There is no authority that can say what yoga is. When you give yourself fully and completely, and experience yoga without limitations or doubts, when you become one with the true experience in yourself, the real encounter with yoga arises. Only then do you understand what yoga is for you. You are no longer limited by ornament, shyness and artificial thought patterns

that lie as a filter between you and the transformation. Yoga is a cultural-historical wealth
that is still passed on from teacher to student
and helps man to find his way back to his true
nature. It opens us up and attracts awareness.
It strengthens our self-esteem, and our entire person's spectrum of possibilities suddenly
becomes visible to us. Yoga is not difficult. You
do not have to be vegan or able to stand on your
head. You just need to practice your yoga regu-
larly and the rest will come by itself.

With all the love from the universe – Om Shanti.

Acharya Shreyananda Natha."

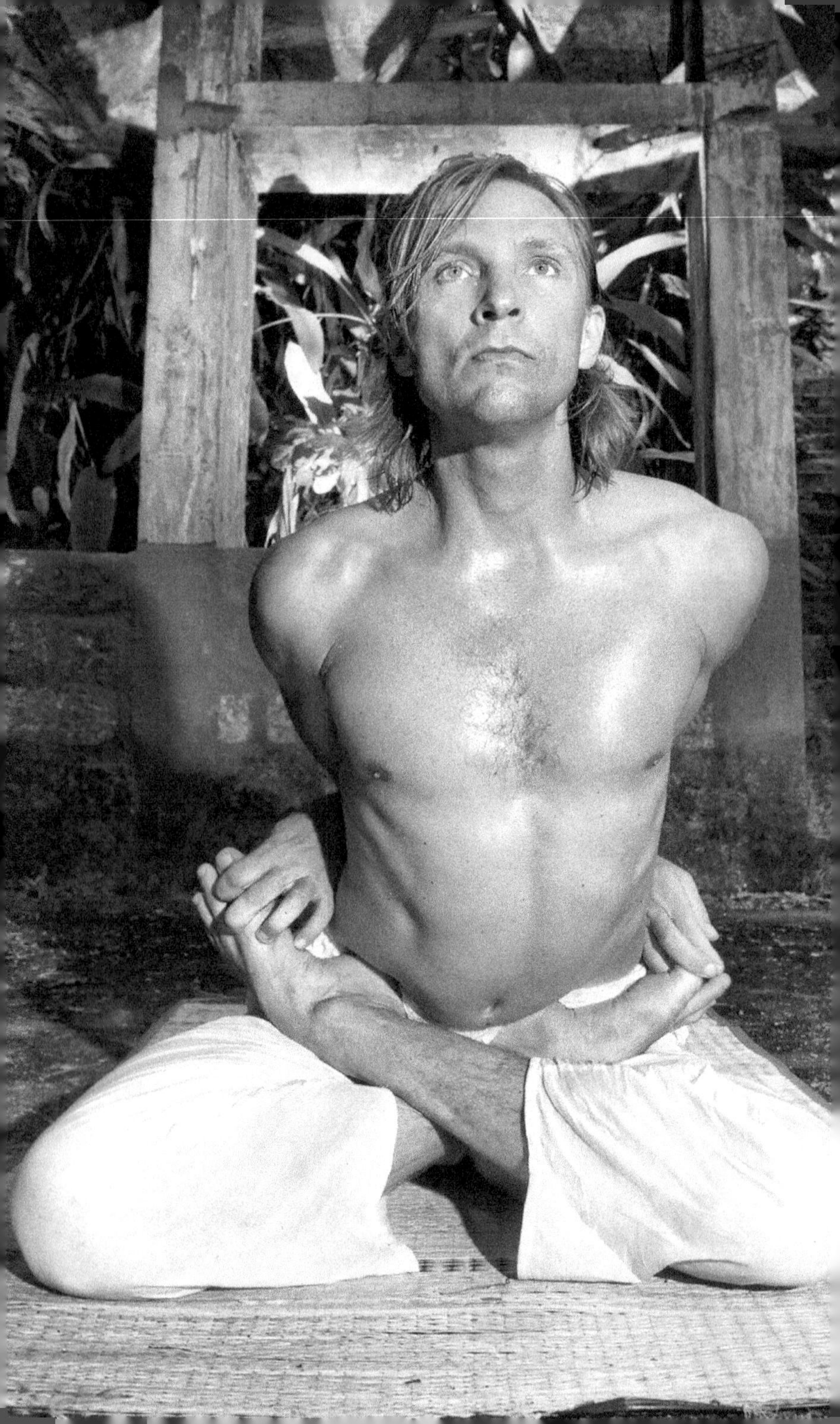

WHAT IS YOGA?

DEFINITION OF YOGA

Yoga chitta vritti nirodha (Yoga Sutras 1.2).
When the mind stills – yoga occurs.

THE MEANING OF YOGA

Yoga means unity and is derived from the word
- yuj, which means to unite in Sanskrit. This
unity or connection in the spiritual sense aims
to unite individual consciousness with universal
consciousness. In practice, this aims to balance
and find harmony between body, mind and emotions. A link between body and soul.

THE PURPOSE OF YOGA

He who knows Kundalini, knows Yoga. The Kundalini, it's said, is coiled like a serpent. He who
can induce her to move is liberated (Hatha Yoga
Pradipika v.105-111).

The absolute purpose of yoga is to awaken
kundalini shakti and make her flow. This is a
precondition for human evolution. Kundalini
shakti flows in the sushi humna nadi along the
spine and activates our most important chakras.
They are in contact with the brain's untapped

resources. When they are used, latent forces are released and we are initiated into the secrets of the universe. We become enlightened and get paranormal abilities – siddhis.

THE GOAL OF YOGA

We can define yoga from a classical perspective; its purpose and meaning, but there is no authority to prescribe what the goal of yoga is – for you. Do you want to reach spiritual goals, get help to rid yourself of back problems or perhaps just be yourself a few minutes a week – free from demands and stress?

There is certainly a big difference in the stated goal of yoga if you practise with aghora sadhus or among orthodox Hindu swamis. Even greater is the difference between Chinese yoga practitioners and atheists in the Americanized ashtanga industry. It is and has always been this way. Thise is the divine essence of yoga. It is as free and amorphous in purpose as in the feeling inside us. Yoga is truly an infinite toolbox. Free to use for what matters most to us. Anandamaya kosha – yoga is unmanifested as our innermost self. When we experience all the power in the universe and on earth – inside and around, we decide for ourselves what the goal of yoga is for us.

THE ORIGIN OF YOGA

The yoga we know today has evolved as part of Tantric civilization. Some believe the first yogi lived about five-thousand years BCE,– others believe that yoga is far older than that.

What we do know is that in the Indus Valley in Harappa and Mohenjodaro (Pakistan), – where the pre-Vedic people once lived around 2600 BCE, statues depicting Shiva and Shakti (Parvati) have been found through archaeological excavations. According to myth, Shiva is the founder of yoga and Parvati is his first disciple. Shiva is seen as a symbol (embodiment) of the highest consciousness. Parvati is considered the mother of the universe. She is the creator and represents knowledge, will, and action. This power, characterized as kundalini shakti, is dormant in every human being. Parvati conveyed the secret knowledge of human liberation through tantra. This is where yoga has its roots and from which it cannot be separated, just as consciousness – (Shiva), cannot be separated from energy – (Shakti).

Yoga probably originated during the beginning of human civilization. Humans began to discover the spiritual potential of man and developed techniques to further develop it. In the past, yoga was kept secret: it was not written down or performed in public. Yoga was passed on orally from guru to student.

Tantric books are the very first to refer to yoga and later also the Vedic scriptures. Rigveda, the oldest Vedic work, was written 3-5000 years BCE, probably by the Indus-Saraswati people. These are a collection of hymns written during the time when the culture in the Indus Valley was still flourishing.

According to legend Shiva (pure consciousness) gave yoga to Parvati (Shakti). A fish overheard their conversation and Shiva turned the fish into a human. Not only animals would have yoga but also humans.

VEDIC YOGA/ARCHAIC YOGA
Dating back to 5000 BCE, Vedic yoga is the oldest form of yoga. Sacrifice was seen as a path to union between inner life, the sensual, and outer life, the material. In order to practice

certain rituals and religions, based on the Vedic hymns (can be compared to the Old Testament), one had to focus and concentrate for an extended period of time. To achieve this, yogic techniques were developed. Today this still remains the basis of yoga; to use inner focus as a way to increase sensory and human abilities.

Vedic yoga was passed on by rishis (seers), not from guru to student.

PRE-CLASSICAL YOGA

Considered an important work between 2000 BCE to 200 years CE, the Upanishads – form part of the Vedic scriptures. The Upanishads consist of two hundred Gnostic texts in which yoga is mentioned. Yoga was now taught from guru to student and used to gain insight.

During this time, there were three important yoga paths:

BHAKTI YOGA – the loving way. It refers to devotion to God or the highest consciousness in any of its manifestations. A loving relationship with God is developed through acts such as singing and reciting the name of God. This is seen as the easiest path to moksha.

JNANA YOGA – the path of knowledge. In Jnana yoga, insight to and understanding of the spiritual aspect is gained by theorizing. Moksha is achieved by understanding that brahman and atman are one and the same.

KARMA YOGA – the path of selfless action. The practice of selfless action unites practition- ers with the highest consciousness. You work and help others without taking credit for it. By being fully present in the work you perform, you become like a tool for the universe.

The Bhagavad Gita, which can be seen as a sum- mary of the Upanishads, takes place on the batt- lefield. Krishna tells Anjuna that by following the three yoga paths he will win the war.

CLASSICAL YOGA

The important work for classical yoga (200CE- 400CE) was Patanjali's Yoga Sutras – a verse book and today, one of the six philosophical paths within Hinduism. Yoga now had its own philosophy. Patanjali divided yoga into eight steps with focus on concentration. In this context, asanas meant a stable and comfor- table position. The physical body was to be steady and immobile during meditation to avoid distraction.

According to Patanjali, an individual is made up of Prakriti (matter) and Purusha (soul). Here, the goal of yoga is to stop identifying with the corporeal body, and in doing so, the soul will be liberated and allowed to reunite with the brahman (universe).

POST-CLASSICAL YOGA

All forms of yoga that came into being after Patanjali are categorized as post-classical yoga (500CE-700CE). Here, tantrism has a great influence. Unlike in classical yoga, the body and the mind were now seen as one. Previously, the body had been experienced as an obstacle, and meditation was used as a means to the body and worldly matters. This era focused on returning to the origin of yoga; to rejuvenate the body and learn to master it in order to awaken kundalini power. According to tantrism, kundalini power exists in every human being, but as a dormant potential. This became the basis of Hatha yoga and the renaissance of tantra. Hatha Yoga Pradipika is an important work in post-classical yoga.

MODERN/CONTEMPORARY YOGA

Swami Vivekananda (1863-1902) was a Hindu theorist and spiritual leader. He was a student of Sri Ramakrishna and founded the Ramakrishna mission in 1897. There they carried out extensive work in healthcare, provided disaster relief and trained people, among other things. In 1898, Vivekananda attended the World's Fair in the United States where he introduced Hinduism which came to play an important role in the invasion of yoga in the West.

Indra Devi (1899-2001), a German yogi, is another person who played an important role in the development of yoga. Indra is seen as the First Lady of yoga. At the time, yoga was primarily studied and practiced by men. Indra was active in the yoga industry for sixty years; she taught many different nationalities and has been a great inspiration to yogis worldwide. Indra was the first to open a yoga studio in the USA in 1947.

Today's most famous tantric yogi is probably the Dalai Lama.

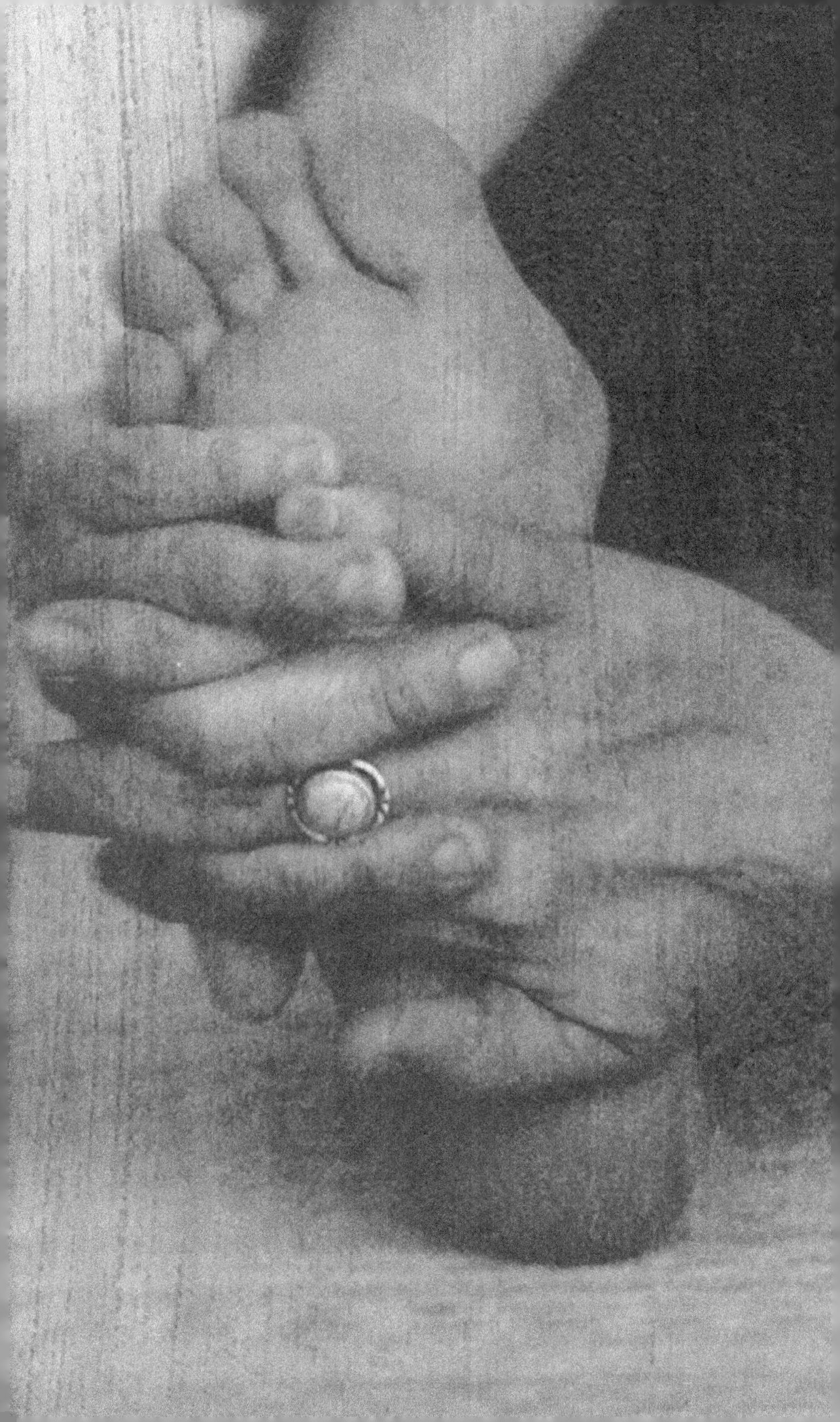

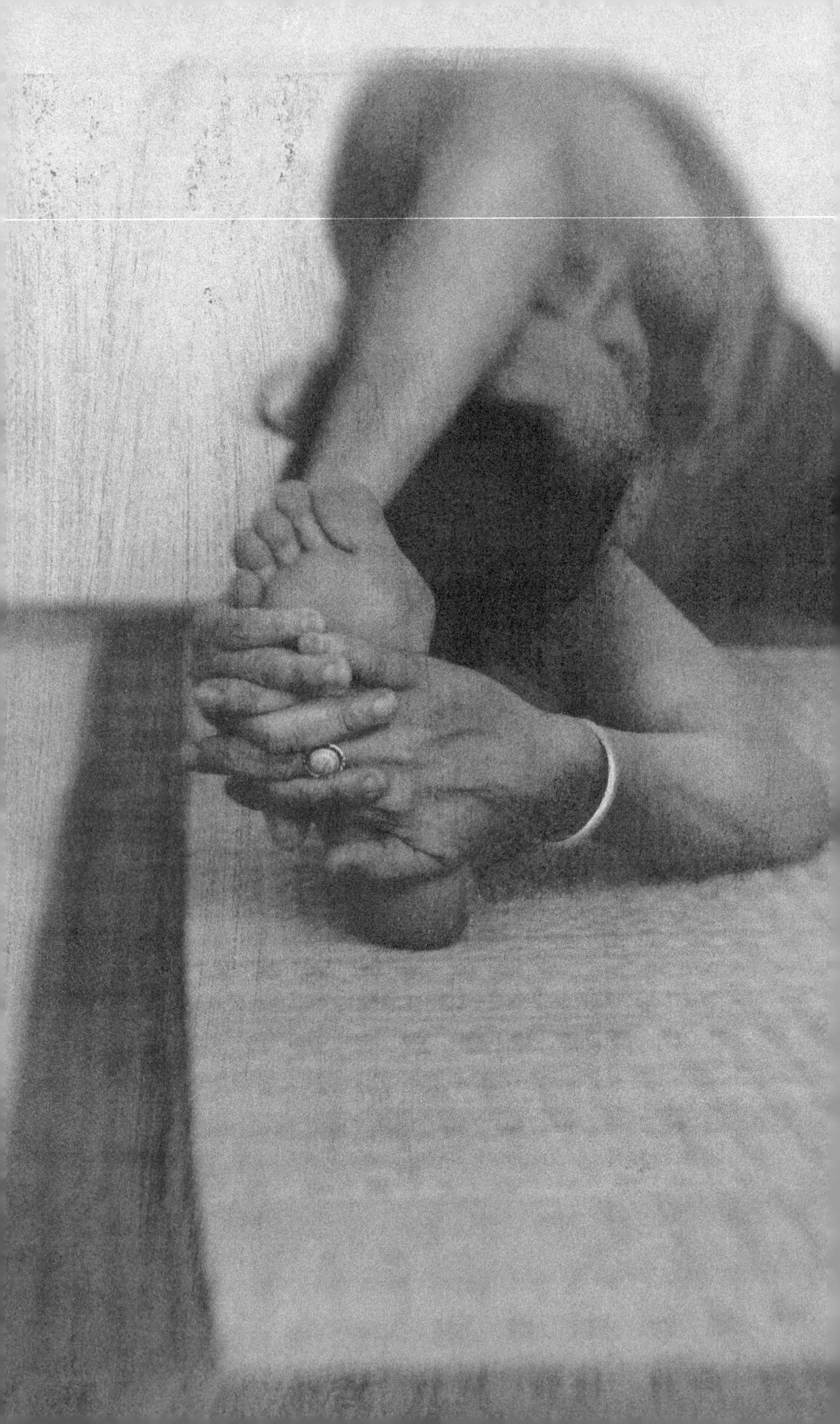

EVOLUTION OF YOGA THROUGH THE 36 TANTRA TATTWAS

36 TANTRA TATTWAS

Man is an image of the universe. The universe is a macrocosm and man is a microcosm. Everything that is created and that we can see, can also be invisible. It comes down to density and goes from the unmanifested to the manifested.

The 36 tantra tattwas describe creation from pure consciousness (Shiva) to matter (Shakti). This is described by 36 steps, 36 manifestations, of energy that go from the fine to the rough.

Everything has its beginning in the macrocosm, where there is pure consciousness. There was a densification of consciousness/energy. A vibration was heard – spandam, the sound of Aum, and thus Shakti was manifested.

"YOU EXPERIENCE ALL POWER
IN COSMOS AND ON EARTH...

IN YOURSELF AND ALL OVER,
EVERYTHING YOU WANT IS POSSIBLE...

BECAUSE ALL POWER IS YOURS."

5 SHIVA TATTWAS
Macrocosmos structure.

SHIVA
The timeless; eternal; space.

SHAKTI
The manifested; time.

ICHA
Will.

JNANA
Knowledge.

KRIYA
Movement.

6 VIDYA TATTWAS

MAYA
Illusion.

KALAA
Contraction of KRIYA.

VIDYA
Contraction of JNANA.

RAGA
Contraction of ICCHA.

KALAA
Contraction of Shakti.

NIYATI – contraction CHICCHAKTI (Shiva).

25 ATMA TATTWAS
Microcosmos; man.

PURUSHA
Shiva.

PRAKRITI
Shakti.

BUDDHI – intellect; insight; SATTVIC GUNA contr. of JNANA.

AHAMKARA – ego; RAJASIC GUNA contraction of ICCHA.

MANAS – thoughts; TAMASIC GUNA contraction of KRIYA.

5 st. JNANENDRIYAS
Sound, touch; sight; taste; smell (sense organs, sattvic).

5 st. KARMENDRIYAS
Speech; feeling; walking, emptying (toilet), sneezing (locomotor system, rajasic).

5 st. TANMANTRA
Sound, taste, shape, smell, touch (sensory attributes, tamasic).

5 st. MAHA BHUTAS
PRITHVI   APAS   AGNI   VAYU   AKASHA
Soil. Water. Fire. Air. Space.

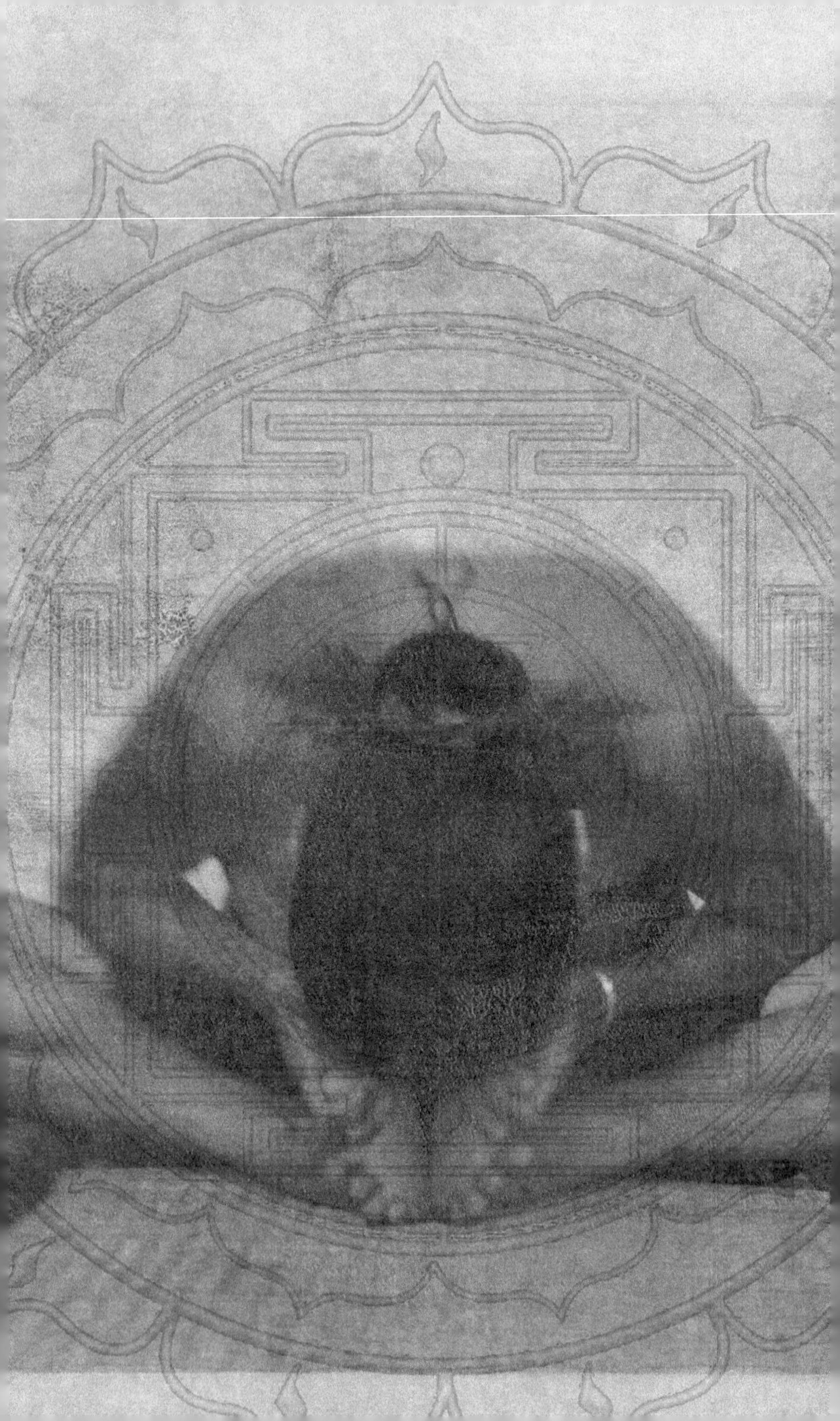

HATHA YOGA

THE BODY CONTROL OF YOGA

A considerable of literature and texts refer to Hatha yoga, most of which were written between 500CE-1400CE of which Hatha Yoga Pradipika by yogi Swatmarama is one of the most famous. References to Hatha yoga are even made in the Upanishads and Puranas, which were written long before the time of Buddhism (about 500 BCE). Traces of Hatha yoga have also been found in pre-Columbian culture in America. Even today there are large stone figures in St. Augustine in South America representing Hatha yoga asanas.

Goraknath, a leading guru in Hatha yoga (approx. 500CE-1100CE). Goraknath was a disciple of Matsyendranatha, the first guru in Hatha yoga. Matsya means fish.

Buddha and Mahavir, the founders of the Jain sect, were two important figures in India around 500BCE. At that time man's spiritual development had been ongoing for centuries.

Two of the Buddha's teachings became known

throughout the world: – Vipassana and Anapa-nasati. For these, the Buddha created a system called the Eightfold Path. This system that deals with ethics and correct livelihood, and it has great similarities to Raja yoga's – yamas and – niyamas. Meditation became a popular method of spiritual development. However, they had no preparatory steps for meditation and eventually began to try the Buddha's system. Meditation was seen as the highest path, but it was acknowledge that some preparations were required before practitioners could sit down to meditate.

Five hundreds years after the time of the Buddha, a Buddhist university was established in Nalanda, Bihar, India. It was called the Hinayana system and was an orthodox Buddhist system.

At the same time, another university was established in Vikram Shila, Bihar, India. It became a learning center espousing the Mahayana tradition. They did not agree with the orthodox interpretation of the Buddha's teachings, viewing the Hinayana system as a deviation from the Buddha's teaching. The Mahayana tradition was founded by a group of liberal Buddhists who

now began to embrace tantric thinking and
philosophy.

After the fall of Buddhism in India (300CE-
500CE, some great yogis wanted to return to
the original doctrine of yoga and tantrism.
Matsyendranatha and Goraknatha were two
of these. They thought that the essence of the
doctrine had been forgotten and misunderstood
by many. They separated Hatha yoga and Raja
yoga from the tantric rituals and developed the
most useful, practical exercises in yoga and
the tantric system. It also became necessary to
reintroduce a proper meditation system. In this
way, Hatha yoga was established. Matsyendranatha founded the Natha order.

To cleanse the body and its elements before
meditation is, the foundation of Hatha yoga.

In Hatha yoga, body and mind are seen as one,
and they are equally important.

THE FIVE ELEMENTS OF HATHA YOGA:

ASANAS
In Raja yoga, asanas refer to a comfortable

and steady position. In Hatha yoga, asanas are specific postures that help to open up our energy channels and energy centers. Hatha yogis discovered that through good body control they also gained control over the mind. Therefore, asanasare put to the forefront in Hatha yoga.

PRANAYAMAS

Breathing is used to influence the flow of prana in our nadis – energy channels. Breathwork is a method through which breathing exercises activate, regulates and purify our life energy in the energy body. You get a higher degree of energy and increase your consciousness.

MUDRAS

Mudra can be translated as posture or gesture. Through mudras, various energy points are stimulated, affecting our body and mind. Mudras can be used to influence your mood, deepen your concentration and consciousness. Through mudras, you hold on to and redirect prana, which would otherwise disappear from the body. In this way, mudras also play an important role in awakening kundalini shakti.

BANDHAS

Traditionally, bandhas are classified as part of mudras. Bandhas are often combined with mudras and pranayamas, but they are an important group of exercises in their own right. Bandha means lock, which describes the exercise and the effect on our energy body. Prana is locked in specific areas of the body and the flow of prana to the sushumna nadi is controlled, which develops our spiritual awakening.

SHATKARMAS

Shatkarmas are a series of purification processes that are divided into six different groups. The purpose of these is to create harmony between ida and pingala nadi in order to achieve mental and physical balance and purity. Purification processes are also used before breathing exercises to expel toxins from the body.

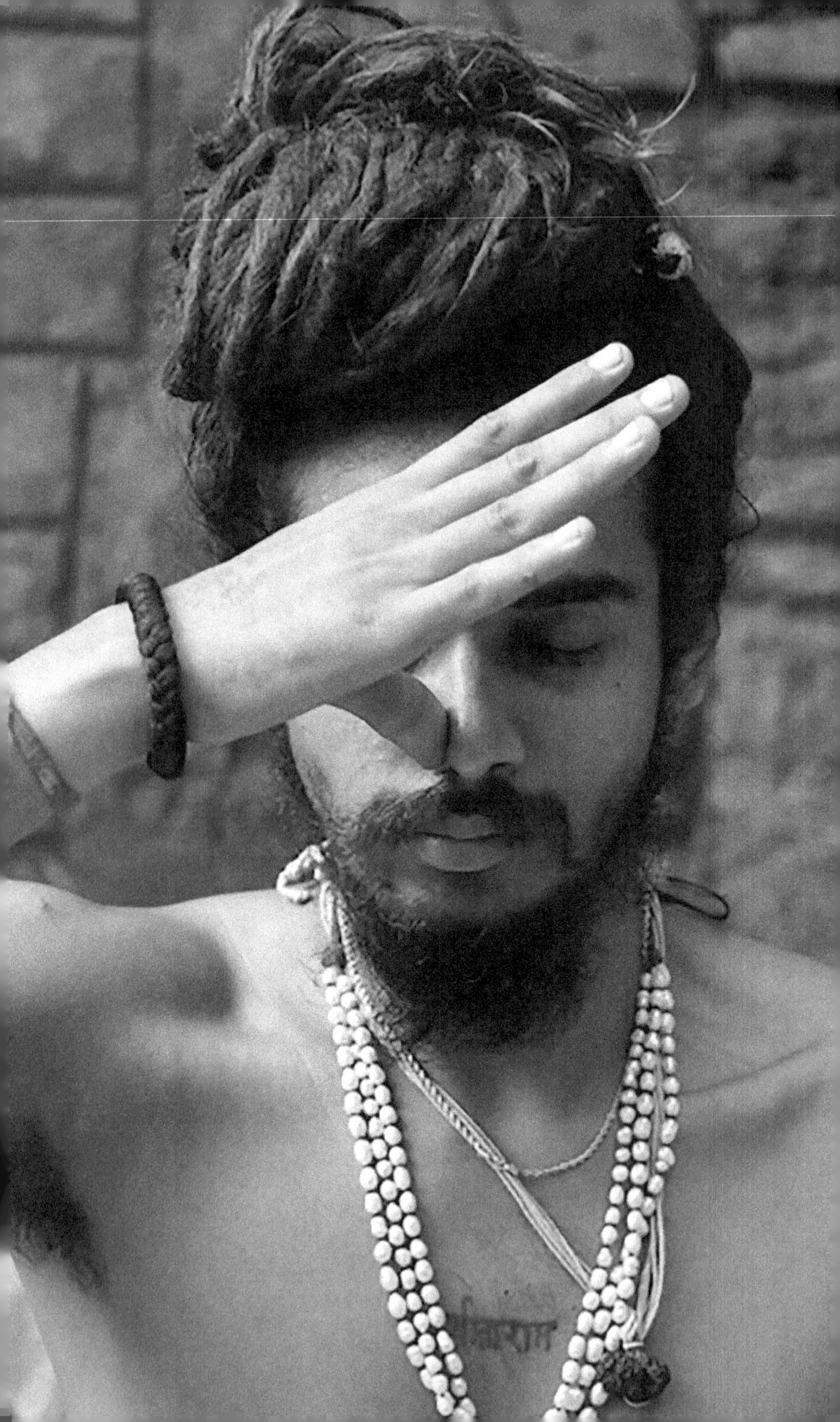

HATHA YOGA PRADIPIKA

Hatha Yoga Pradipika is a classic textbook in Hatha yoga. It was written in the fifteenth century by Svami Svatmarama who was a disciple of Svami Gorakhnatha. Hatha Yoga Pradipika is thus the oldest preserved Hatha yoga text and one of the three classical texts, next to Gheranda Samhita and Shiva Samhita.

The book contains a total of three-hundred and ninety verses. Of these, about forty are dedicated to asanas, about one-hundred to pranayamas, one-hundred and fifty to mudras, bandhas and shatkarmas, and the rest to pratyahara, dharana, dhyana and samadhi. The book consists of four chapters:

1.) Asana: Svatmarama honors his teachers, explains why he wrote the book and who he wrote it for. He describes how and where yoga should be practiced. Svatmarama then describes fifteen asanas and gives recommendations for eating habits.

2.) Pranayama: Svatmarama addresses the connections between breathing, mind, kundalini, bandha, nadi and prana. He then describes six karmas and eight kumbhakas.

3.) Mudras: The author describes ten different mudras.

4.) Samadhi: Svatmarama discusses samadhi, laya, nada, two mudras and the four steps of yoga.

Hatha Yoga Pradipika is dedicated to Lord Adi-natha, which is another name for Shiva (a Hindu god of destruction and renewal), is believed to have revealed the mysteries of Hatha yoga to his divine consort Parvati.

HE WHO KNOWS KUNDALINI, KNOWS
YOGA.

THE KUNDALINI, IT'S SAID,
IS COILED LIKE A SERPENT.

HE WHO CAN INDUCE HER TO MOVE
IS LIBERATED.

(HATHA YOGA PRADIPIKA V.105-111)

HATHA YOGA

OUR FIVE SHEATHS
Our physical body, the three bodies of the astral body and our innermost interior.

Hatha yoga teaches that we consist of five sheaths or bodies:

ANNAMAYA KOSHA
Physical body.

PRANAMAYA KOSHA
Energy body.

MANAMAYA KOSHA
Mental body.

VIGYANAMAYA KOSHA
Wisdom body.

ANANDAMAYA KOSHA
Blissbody (pure consciousness of true self).

The energy body, the mental body and the wisdom body form the astral body.

NADIS – IDA AND PINGALA AND SUSHUMNA NADI

Pranamaya kosha – our energy body, consists of about seventy-two-thousand nadis (subtle channels through which prana flows). It is the energy body that gives us life. The three most important nadis are ida, pingala and sushumna nadi of which sushumna nadi is the most important.

Ida nadi flows from the left side of the spine and controls mental energy. It is associated with the parasympathetic nervous system. Pingala nadi flows along the right side of the spine and controls our physical body. It is associated with the sympathetic nervous system. Sushumna nadi, the most important of the three, flows along the entire spine and channels the spiritual energy.

Ida and pingala nadi flow from the root chakra and cross the sushumna nadi at four places in the body to finally unite at the eyebrow center. Ida nadi then goes out through the left nostril and pingala nadi through the right.

We can regulate the body's energies through asanas, and when ida and pingala nadi flow simultaneously, sushumna nadi opens. Kundalini shakti can begin to travel upwards and activate our chakra system, thereby illuminating the parts of our brain that are dormant. Usually, we use about twenty percent of our brain capacity. On our path to activating a larger part of the brain, special siddhis, – paranormal abilities, arise. You become a siddha. However, these abilities are not the ultimate goal.

HA+THA

Ha – pingala nadi – the sun, stands for the sympathetic nervous system, and tha – ida nadi – the moon, stands for the parasympathetic nervous system.

OUR SUBTLE ENERGY BODY WITH FIVE PRANA VAYUS

Our five bodies interact with each other and create a whole. The breathing exercises mainly affect our energy body, – pranamaya kosha, which is made up of five different types of sub-pranas. These five prana vayus (wind) are: prana, apana, samana, udana and vyana. It is also the link that binds the bodies together and affects us in all directions. If we calm the body with breathing, we also calm the mind and vice versa, which you probably have experienced during your yoga practice.

PRANA

In this context, prana does not refer to the cosmic prana, but to the flow of energy that controls the area of the thorax between the larynx and the diaphragm. This area is linked to the heart and respiratory system along with the muscles and nerves that activate them. It is this power that makes us draw inward breath.

APANA

Apana controls the abdomen, and the area under the navel, and it provides energy to the intestines, kidneys, rectum and genitals. It affects the expulsion of waste products in the body and is the force that makes us exhale.

SAMANA

Samana is located between the heart and the navel. It activates and controls the digestive system. Samana is responsible for the transformation: physically, the transformation refers to the very distribution of nutrients in the body, and evolutionarily, it refers to kundalini power and the development of our consciousness.

UDANA

Udana controls the area of the neck and head. It activates all our sensory receptors such as eyes, tongue, nose and ears. Udana activates and creates a balance in muscles, ligaments, nerves and joints in our arms and legs. It is responsible for our posture, our sensory attention and our ability to interact with the outside world.

VYANA

Vyana permeates the whole body. It regulates and controls all our movements and coordinates all sub-pranas in the body.

In addition to the most important sub-pranas, there are also five smaller pranas called upa-pranas. These five are naga, koorma, krikara, devadatta and dhananjaya. Naga is responsible for belching and hiccups, koorma opens our eyes and makes us blink, krikara creates hunger, thirst, sneezing and coughing, devadatta generates sleep and yawning, and dhananjaya activates when we die and our body begins to break down.

PRANA AND LIFESTYLE

Our lifestyle has a big impact on our energy

body and its prana. Physical activity such as exercise, work, sleep, food and sexual relationships affect the distribution and flow of prana in our body. Emotions, thoughts and fantasies affect our body even more. An unbalanced lifestyle, poor diet and stress break down and block the flow of prana. It results in feeling drained of energy. When energy becomes low in one of our sub-pranas, the very area of the body that the prana controls is affected and may result in illness. Breathing exercises can prevent this by balancing or increasing the energy in our energy body.

ASANA

There is a definition of asanas – Stirham Sukham Asana in Patanjali's Yoga Sutras, which means steady or comfortable position. They wanted to develop their ability to sit still for a long time, because it was a prerequisite for meditation.

In Hatha yoga, however, it was discovered that certain postures – asanas, opened up energy channels and mental centers in the body. You got better body control and could thus also develop control over the mind, thoughts, and energies. Yoga asanas became a tool for achieving a higher consciousness and provided the stable foundation required to explore the body, mind and breathing.

Originally, there were eight-million-four-hund-red-thousand different asanas. These represent as many lives as an unenlightened person must be reborn into before he becomes enlightened. Rishis and yogis scaled down the number to the few hundred known today. Of these, the eighty-four most important asanas were then produced. There are thirty-five asanas that have a direct impact on our chakras. The others purify and regulate our nadis. Asanas create a balance between body and mind and a flow in the sushumna.

Rishis studied the animals and notice how they lived in harmony with their body and surroundings. By mimicking the animals movements and postures, hormone secretion in the body was affected. During deep meditation, they were able to observe how different postures affected both the body and the mind.

Prana, the vital energy (life energy), permeates

our entire body. Poor flow of prana in the body results in stiffness and an accumulation of toxins. When prana flows freely, these toxins are removed and the body becomes soft and supple. Even the most difficult postures are easy to perform. When the amount of prana increases in the body, "pranic intuition" is achieved. An inutive sense of how to perform asanas, mudras and pranayamas follows.

Hatha yoga not only increases overall health but also activates our energy centers by balancing the nervous system.

Asanas in Hatha yoga release tensions that arise as knots in our muscles. By releasing these tensions from the body, we also release tensions from the mind. It makes us feel better in general and releases underlying and hidden energy that lies latent.

Thus asanas are more than just exercise. They are techniques that place the body in different positions to promote awareness, relaxation, concentration and meditation. Part of this process is to develop a good physique through stretching, stimulation of prana, and massage of the glands and internal organs.

Asanas are divided into three groups: – beginners, intermediate and advanced. It is not necessary to complete all the exercises in each group. Daily practice of a tailor-made program will have the greatest effect.

Asanas for beginners should be performed by those who have never practiced yoga before. These have a greater effect on the body in beginners than advanced exercises. These exercises prepare the body and mind for the more advanced exercises as well as meditation and are very useful for improving physical health.

The intermediate asanas, are for those who can complete the exercises for beginners without difficulty. These require greater concentration, steadiness and coordination in connection with movement and breathing.

Advanced asanas are for those who have well-developed body control, muscles and nervous system. You should be able to master the intermediate exercises without problem. It is important not to rush and start these exercises too early.

DYNAMIC AND STATIC ASANAS

Dynamic asanas increase flexibility and circulation in the body. They soften muscles, release knots and energy blockages, and remove stagnant blood. These asanas are most important for the beginner. To be able to work with the chakra system for example, blockages must first be released, otherwise the energy may flow the wrong way in the energy body. Dynamic asanas and vinyasan process our physical body: they take us deeper and prepare us for the more static asanas. Hatha yoga often starts with a lot of movement and then gradually lets the vibrations subside into stillness and silence. This also has a lot to do with us moving from the rough to the fine – from the body to the mind –, and the knowledge of how yoga affects our doshas through Ayurveda.

VINYASA

Dynamic asanas are often synchronized with breathing. When we do that, it's called vinyasa. A flow where movements and breathing interact.

Vinyasa aims to increase the internal cleansing and detoxification of the body. Breathing synchronized with movement warms the blood. Thick blood is often unhealthy and causes diseases. The heat from vinyasa cleanses the blood and makes it thinner so it can circulate better in the body, around our joints and reduce any pain.

Where there is poor circulation in the body, pain usually occurs. The heated blood also passes through all the internal organs, and transports impurities and diseases away that are removed from the body with our increased amount of sweat during the yoga session.

Sweat is an important by-product of vinyasa. It is only through our sweat that diseases can leave the body and be purified, in the same way that gold is melted to get rid of its impurities. Yoga boils the blood and transports impurities and toxins to the surface, which are then removed with the help of sweat. If you practice vinyasa often, the body becomes healthy and strong, and clean and shiny like gold.

With the body cleansed, it is possible to cleanse the nervous system and sense organs.

STATIC ASANAS

Static and, above all inverted asanas have the deepest effect on our energy body and our chakra system. These require greater flexibility and are suited for the more experienced practitioners. To remain in the position for a few minutes, gives a more powerful effect on the glands, prana, chakras and internal organs. The mind becomes calm and prepares the individual for meditation. Some static asanas are very useful for reaching pratyahara.

TRISTHANA

Tristhana means three areas to pay attention to: postures (position, stretching and relaxation), breath and gazing point. They are always performed in conjunction with each other.

Asanas cleanse, strengthen and soften the body. When we breathe with rechaka and puraka, a steady and even inhalation and exhalation at the same pace, we cleanse the nervous system. Drishti is the place you look at during yoga practice. There are nine different ones: tip of the nose, eyebrow center, navel, thumbs, hands, feet, right and left side, up to the sky. Drishi purifies, captures and stabilizes the mind.

ADVICE FOR THE PRACTICE OF ASANAS:
BREATH

According to Hatha yoga, two components
are needed to cleanse the body internally: the
elements air and fire. Fire, – our life force, is
located at the solar plexus in the body and is ge-
nerated by the Manipura chakra. Air is required
for fire to burn, hence the importance of proper
breathing in yoga. Long, even breaths increase
the internal fire, – agnin in the body, which in
turn heats up the blood for physical purification
and burns up impurities in the nervous system.
As the internal fire increases in strength, so
does our digestive system, health and longevity.
Uneven breathing creates an imbalance in both
our physical body and, its signaling system,
weakening our immune system. We risk beco-
ming ill in the long run – according to Hatha
yoga, we tolerate both stress and toxins less.

Another important component to increase the
inner fire is to use moola and uddiyana bandha:
root and stomach locks. They increase the effect
of breathing, keep it inside the body longer,
encapsulate the energy, and provide light, strength and health to the body.

According to Hatha yoga, there are six toxins
in the body that surround our spiritual heart.
The light in our hearts is obscured by these six
poisons: kama, krodha, moha, lobha, matsa-
rya, and mada. These are lust, anger, delusion,
greed, envy and sloth. When we have practiced
Hatha yoga for an extended period of time with
power, determination and the right breathing,
the increasing heat in the body will burn up
these six toxins and the light in our interior will
shine through.

It is important to breathe through the nose
(unless otherwise stated) and coordinate breathing with the movement. But never force
yourself to breathe through your nose. If you
need to breathe through your mouth, do it. Your
fine energy channels can be damaged otherwise
and the energy will flow the wrong way in the
energy body. If you are panting, wait until you
can breathe through your nose again without it
greater difficulty.

CONSCIOUSNESS

The purpose of asanas is to influence and create
harmony in all aspects of man: physical, mental, emotional, pranic and spiritual. By perfor-

ming asanas consciously, all these parts are affected. One should be aware of body sensations, movement, posture on its own and in coordination with breathing, the flow of prana, focus on chakra and witness thoughts and feelings that come up.

RELAXATION

You can lie down in shavasana at any time for rest or contemplation. Notice how it feels in the body.

SERIES

You always begins with shatkarmas (purification processes) such as nasal rinsing (jala neti), – then you perform asanas, pranayamas, pratyahara and dharana (concentration quiet the mind) which lead to dhyana (meditation). You can also add both breathing exercises and meditation before asanas. It fulfills a function – especially at the beginning of your yoga practice, that you go from the outside in (see the text about our five bodies) before you intuitively know what, when and how to do.

OPPOSITION

It is important to have a structure in the pro-

gram to balance the body and nervous system.
A forward bending position should always be
followed by a backward bending position and
vice versa. However, this does not apply to yoga
rehabilitation.

TIME

Asanas can be practiced at any time of the day,
provided you have not eaten a few hours prior.
With that said, it is recommended to practice
just before sunrise and sunset. The time of day
just before sunrise is called Brahmamuhurta (the
divine time – God's time). The atmosphere is
clean and still then, the stomach and intestines
inactive and the mind still. The most favorable
time is before sunrise and before sunset, but do
not be too ambitious from the outset. It is better
to have a yoga session during the day, than no
session at all.

PLACE

One should find a secluded place where it is
tidy, clean, quiet and peaceful. No furniture
or objects should be in the way. You can also
practice outdoors in a comfortable and beautiful
place. However, not in the cold and wind, or
where the air is unclean or in scorching sun.

CARPET

Use a base of natural materials. It has the most beneficial effect on our pranic currents.

CLOTHES

Wear loose and comfortable clothes, and remove jewelry, and be barefoot so you do not slip.

SHOWER

Try to take a cold shower before the session to wake the body up. After the session, wait to shower so you do not cool down your body too quickly and lose the healing effect of yoga unnecessarily.

LOO

Empty the stomach.

DIET

There are no strict rules regulating what food to eat. However, a natural diet in moderate amounts is recommended so that not all energy is used to digest food. A vegetarian diet is not essential but it is recommended. The stomach should be filled half with food, a quarter with water and a quarter should be left empty. However, do not drink water during the practice as it draws blood and energy to the stomach and cools down your energy body. As you know, we want to get the energy out of the body during yoga. Also, wait two to three hours to practice yoga after you have eaten so it does not feel uncomfortable during the session.

PERFORMANCE

Asanas are performed softly and gently in three steps:

Awareness of the body, movement and thoughts that arise. This creates calm, balance and focus, which in turn leads to a state of harmony in the body.

Awareness of breathing. Synchronize movement with breathing. The movement becomes calmer and brain waves slower. You become relaxed and gain an increased awareness.

Awareness of the flow of prana. It can be experienced as tingles in the body. The feeling is developed through regular practice. You become mentally calm, focused, and emotionally receptive.

Asanas are also divided into three parts:

Starting poses.
Implementation.
Final poses.

IMPORTANT

In the event of any injury or illness, a physician should be consulted before performing asanas.

Asanas must never hurt joints, hard parts or ligaments during practice.

Inverted asanas should be avoided during gas formation (toxins can reach the brain), late pregnancy, and menstruation (the cycle can be disrupted). Never sunbathe immediately fol-lowing yoga practice to avoid overheating.

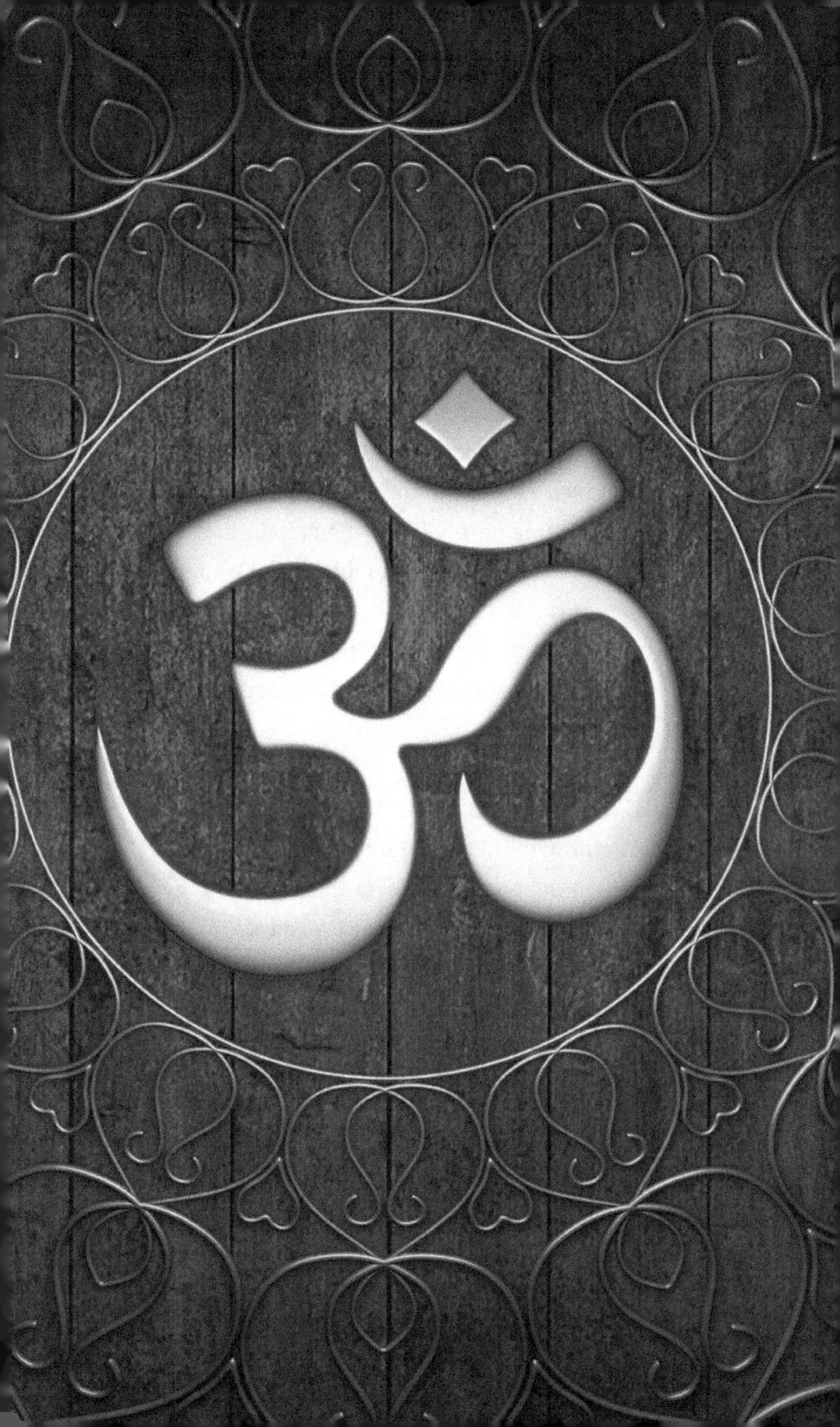

PRANAYAMA

Pranayama means breathing technique or breathing control, and originates from the words: prana (life force or life energy), yama (discipline or control) and ayama (extension, restraint or expansion). Pranayamas are divided into puraka (inhalation), kumbhaka (retention of breath), and rechaka (exhalation). Kumbhaka, in turn, is divided into antar and bahir (the retention of breath immediately following exhalation). In yogic writings, kevala kumbhaka is also mentioned. It is an advanced yogic condition where breathing via the lungs stops spontaneously and energy (prana) seeps through the pores in the body's cells.

HEALTH AND BREATHING

Breathing is the most important function we have in the body. It affects the activity of every single cell, including the brain and its functions. A person breathes about fifteen breaths per minute and about twenty-thousand-six-hundred breaths per day. Most of us breathe incompletely, using only a small part of our lungs' capacity. The breathing then becomes shallow and the body becomes poor in oxygen and prana, which are necessary to maintain good health.

Rhythmic, deep and slow breathing encoura-
ges and is encouraged by a calm and satisfied
state of mind. Irregular and uneven breathing
disrupts the rhythm of the brain, which leads
to physical, emotional, and mental blockages.
This, in turn, cause internal conflicts, an unbalanced personality, a disordered lifestyle, and
illness. Through the breathing exercises, you
build up a regular breathing pattern and break
this vicious circle. We learn to regain control of
our breathing and rebuild the natural, relaxed
rhythm of our body and mind.

Despite being an unconscious process, you can
turn breathing into a conscious process at any
time. This creates a link between the unconscious and the conscious parts of our mind. The
energy that is absorb by neurotic and unconscious mental patterns can be released with the help
of breathing exercises. The energy can then be
used on something creative and joyful.

BREATHING AND LIFE
Ancient yogis and rishis studied nature in detail.
They noted that animals with slow breathing
had a long lifespan and animals with fast
breathing only lived for a few years. Through

this observation, they realized how important slow breathing is for a longevity. Physically, breathing is directly linked to the heart. Slow breathing keeps the heart strong which leads to a longer life. Deep breathing also increases the absorption of energy in our energy body, which increases mobility, vitality and our well-being.

BREATHING EXERCISES AND THE SPIRITUAL SEARCH

Breathing exercises build a healthy body by releasing blockages in the energy body, this increases the absorption and retention of pran in the body. A calm and quiet mind is a prerequisite for spiritual exercises. In many breathing exercises, kumbhaka (retention of breath) is used to control the flow of prana, calm the mind, and control the thought process. When the mind is calmed down and prana can flow freely through our nadis and chakras, the development of our consciousness is enabled. This in turn can lead us to higher dimensions of spiritual experiences.

COMMON ADVICE

Contraindications. Breathing exercises should not be practiced during illness. However, lighter exercises such as conscious breathing or abdominal breathing in shavasana are still acceptable.

TIME

The best time for breathing exercises is in the morning before the sun rises. The body is calm and the mind still as it has not yet had time to absorb many impressions from its surroundings. If this is not possible, the second-best time is in the evening when the sun goes down. Soothing breathing exercises are good to do before falling asleep. Try to do the breathing exercises at the same time and in the same place every day. Regular practice builds strength and willpower.

HYGIENE

Take a bath or shower before practicing pranayamas. At least, wash hands, face and feet. Wait at least half an hour to bathe after completing breathing exercises. This is to allow the body temperature to normalize.

FOOD

Eat your breakfast after completing the practice or wait three to four hours after eating to practice. With food in the stomach, a pressure is formed on the diaphragm and lungs, which makes it difficult to breathe deeply and completely. It hinders the use of full capacity of the lungs.

When you start practicing breathing exercises, you may experience constipation and a decrease in urine. If this occurs, reduce salt and spices, and drink plenty of water. Should you instead experience an anxious stomach and an increase in urine take a break from practice for a few days.

PLACE

Practice in a place where you can find peace and quiet, and where it is clean. The place should be well ventilated, but not so that you are sitting in a draft. Avoid direct sunlight as it may cause overheating.

BREATH

Always breathe through your nose unless otherwise instructed. The air must be able to flow freely through both nostrils.

SEQUENCE

Breathing exercises are done after shatkarmas and often after asanas, and before meditation, but can also be practiced before asanas. Nadi shodana should be included in each breathing exercise. Lie down in shavasana for a few minutes after completing the exercises.

SITTING POSITION

A comfortable sitting position is necessary to be able to keep the body and breathing stable during the exercises. The body should be as relaxed as possible with a straight spine and neck. The seat pad should be made of natural material. If you can not sit comfortably in a meditation position for a long time, you can sit against a wall with outstretched legs or on a chair with a straight backrest.

Avoid exertion. It is important to remember not to exert too much effort when doing breathing exercises. Do not be in a hurry to advance. Do not move on to the next step until you feel fully comfortable with an exercise. Keeping your breath inside/out is only achieved as long as it feels comfortable.

SIDE EFFECTS

Various physical and mental symptoms can occur in normally healthy people. Physical symptoms occur as a result of the detoxification of toxins. Feelings such as tingling, heat and cold, lightness and heaviness may occur. These are usually temporary. Energy levels may increase or fluctuate and interests may change. If these changes create problems, you should seek the guidance of a competent guru. Excessive pranayamas late at night can lead to sleeping problems as well as an extreme excess of energy the next day – what many describe as a kundalini awakening, or hypersensitivity. Pranayamas are powerful tools and should be treated with respect. Slightly simplified, you can say that through breathing exercises agni (fire) is increased in us, and manipura chakra at the navel increases its activity. This causes vayu (air) attached to the chakra above, anahata, to be netted and expanded. As the air expands, so does the space within us (akasha) and a deeper spiritual experience is reached. However, increasing the amount of vayu can lead to anxiety and worry, so it is important that you end each session by reducing the excess of vata you have built up.

MUDRA/HOLDING

Mudra can be translated as "posture" or "gesture". Through mudras, various energy points that

affect both body and mind are stimulated. Your
mood is influenced and your consciousness and
ability to concentrate are increased. With the
help of mudras, you can hold and control prana
that would otherwise disappear from the body.
Hence, mudras also play an important role in
awakening kundalini energy. Mudras can be
done as a single exercise or in combination with
asanas, pranayamas, bandhas and different
visualization techniques.

In Hatha Yoga Pradipika, mudras are discussed
as "yoganaga": a separate branch of yoga that
requires a subtle presence. You often learn these
techniques after you have become accustomed
to and knowledgeable in asanas, pranayamas,
bandhas and when you have eliminated blockages from the body. Mudras are among the more
advanced techniques that awaken our prana,
chakra and kundalini shakti, which in turn can
open up various siddhis (paranormal or mental
forces) in the more advanced practitioners.

Mudras create a direct link between annamaya
kosha (our physical body), manomaya kosha (our
mental body) and pranamaya kosha (our energy
body). This increases the feeling and awareness

of the flow of prana in the body. A pranic balance is created in our koshas and the subtle energy is directed to the higher chakras, which promotes an increased degree of consciousness.

Our nadis and chakras radiate energy, which normally disappears from the body into our surroundings. By creating barriers within the body with the help of mudras, the energy is instead directed inwards. According to Tantric literature, when prana is kept in the body with the help of mudras, the mind becomes introverted, which leads to pratyahara, – withdrawal of our senses, as well as dharana (concentration).

Mudras can be divided into five different categories:

HASTA/HAND MUDRA
These lead the energy created in our hands back into the body. You create an energy path that flows from the brain to the hands and then back again. If you are aware of this process, an inner awareness is created quickly.

Mudras in this category are: jnana mudra, chin mudra, yoni mudra, bhairava mudra, and hridayamudra.

MANA/HEAD MUDRA

These techniques are an important part of kundalini yoga and many are used as meditation techniques. Here you use eyes, ears, nose, tongue and lips.

Mudras in this category are: shambavi mudra, nasikagra drishti, khechari mudra, khaki mudra, bhujangini mudra, bhoochari mudra, akashi mudra, shanmukhi mudra, and unmani mudra.

KAYA MUDRA

These exercises are combined with asanas, breathing techniques and concentration.

Mudras in this category are: vipareeta karani mudra, pashinee mudra, prana mudra, yoga mudra, manduki mudra, and tadagi mudra.

BANDHA/LOCK

These exercises combine mudras and bandhas. They charge the system with prana and prepare for the awakening of kundalini shakti.

Techniques in this category are: maha mudra, maha bheda mudra, and maha vedha mudra.

Adhara: – these techniques direct the prana from lower parts of the body to the brain.
Techniques that use sexual energy belong to this
group and are extremely powerful.

Techniques in this category are: ashwini mudra
and varjoli/sahajoli mudra.

MUDRAS AND OUR ELEMENTS

In the yogic tradition, our hands are like a map
of our well-being. Different points in our hands
are directly linked to other body parts and our
psyche. By making different mudras or hand
positions, we stimulate these points and energy
paths.

Our physical body, like our surroundings, is
made up of five different elements: earth,
water, fire, air and ether (space). Many people
know the first four elements, but ether (space)
is often unknown. Ether (space) is a subtle energy, a celestial energy that exists high above our
earth. In our body, ether is the space within us
at cellular level.

Imbalances in our elements weaken our immune
system which in the long run leads to illness.

These deficiencies or imbalances can be corrected by connecting different parts of the body to each other in a specific way precisely by mudras. Mudras create electromagnetic currents in the body, so-called energy loops. Each element is also associated with a chakra. When the element is balanced, the chakra is also affected and in turn affects the energy (vayu) that belongs to the chakra's area.

Finger: Element/tattwa; chakra; energi/vayu.

Thumb: Fire/agni; Manipura; Samana.

Index finger: Air/vayu; Anahata; Prana.

Middle finger: Ether/akasha; Vishuddhi; Udana.

The ring finger: Earth/prithvi; Mooladhara; Apana.

Little finger: Water/apas; Swadhistana; Vyana.

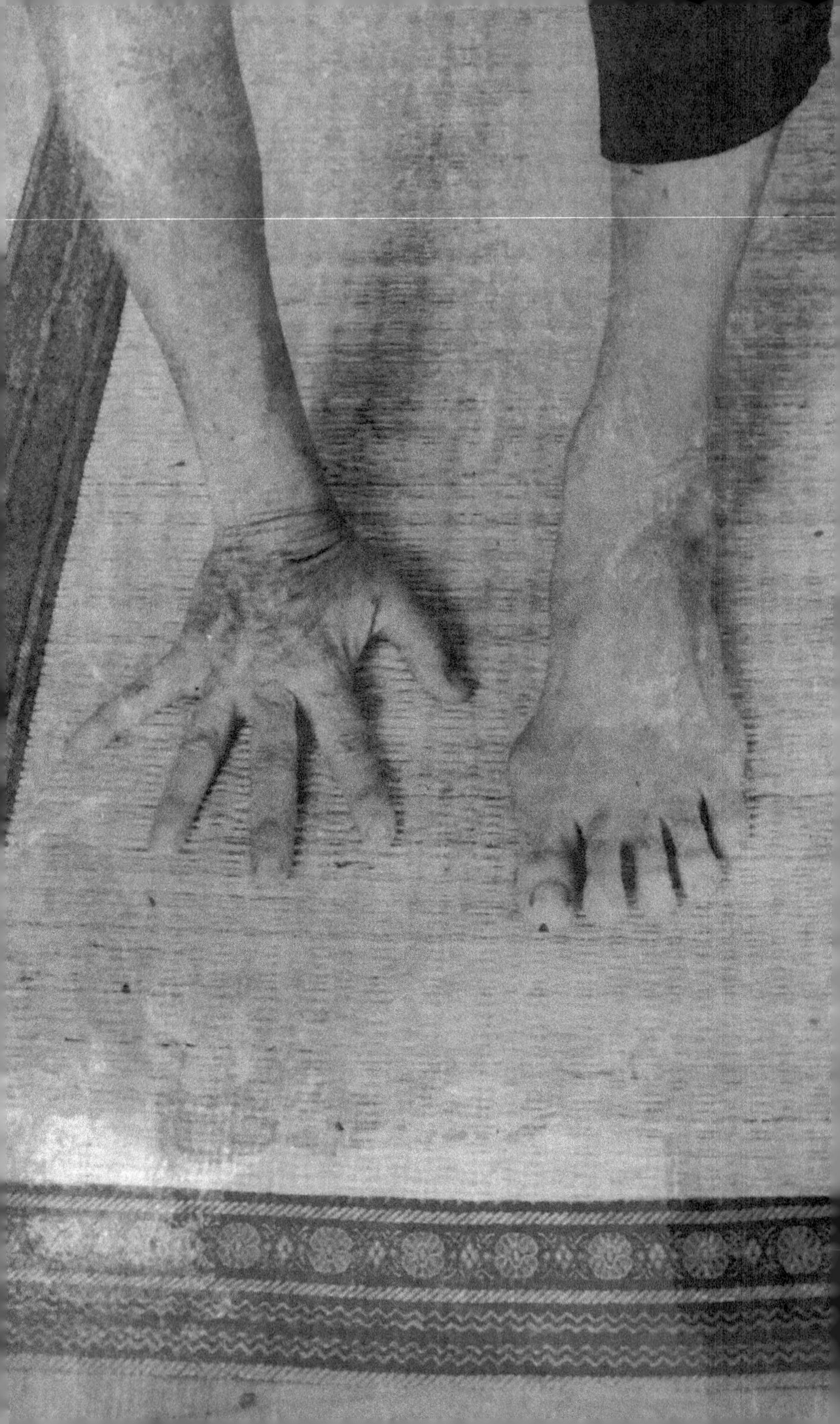

HASTA MUDRA PRANAYAMA

(4 four steps)

SEQUENCE

1. Chin mudra pranayama.

Sit in a comfortable meditation position. Extend the spine and neck. Place your hands, palm facing up,on your knees. Press your thumb against the index finger and let the other fingers point straight out. Sit still, close your eyes and follow your natural breathing for a few minutes.

Chin mudra opens up the lower lobes of the lungs and stimulates apana vayu (prana that moves down from the navel to the perineum). Physically, it is responsible for the expulsion of toxins in the body.

Sit still and follow the breathing that moves in and out of the nose. Two to three minutes.

2. Chin maya mudra pranayama.

Now fold in your fingers without touching your palms. Hold your thumb against your index finger.

Chin maya mudra pranayama opens up the middle lobes

of our lungs and stimulates the samana vayu (prana that moves from left to right in the area around the abdomen). Physically, it is responsible for digestion and our ability to assimilate the nutrients in our food. On a subtle level, it affects our ability to absorb (and learn from) experiences in our life.

Sit still and follow the breathing that moves in and out of the nose. Two to three minutes.

3. Aadi mudra pranayama.

Now grab the thumbs with other your fingers and place the fists on the knees with the back of the hand up.

Aadi mudra pranayama opens the upper lobes of our lungs. It stimulates the udana vayu (prana that moves upwards towards the head and outwards in our extremities). Physically, it is responsible for healing and balancing our sense organs. On a subtle level, it is responsible for balancing our perception.

Sit still and follow the breathing that moves in and out of the nose. Two to three minutes.

4. Brahma mudra pranayama.

Hold the position of the hands, but turn them so that the wrists are facing upwards and the knuckles are facing each other. Press your hands against your body level with your pelvis.

Brahma mudra pranayama opens up the whole lung. It opens up vyana vayu – the energy that makes us go on a bit longer, "the last boost". It balances and starts our other pranas in the body when they become low. It revitalizes the whole system. Sit still and follow the breathing that moves in and out of the nose. Two to three minutes.

BANDHA AND GRANTHI/LOCKS AND BLOCK-ING

Traditionally, bandhas are classified as part of mudras. In Hatha Yoga Pradipika and in old tantric texts, mudras and bandhas are seen as a whole, they are not separated. Bandhas are linked to mudras and to pranayamas. Bandhas are a technique that create a unique lock in the body.

The word bandha means "to hold" or "lock" in

Sanskrit. It describes the physical effect created in the body and the retention of prana. Bandhas lock the energy into specific parts of the body and control the flow to the sushumna nadi in order to create a spiritual awakening.

Bandhas should be learn as a separate technique before practicing them together with mudras and pranayamas.

There are four different "locking techniques": jalandhara, moola, uddiyana and maha bandha. Maha is a combination of the first three. These three bandhas have a direct impact on our three mental points (granthis) in the body. Moola bandha is associated with brahma granthi, uddiana bandha with vishnu granthi and jalandhara bandha with rudra granthi. Granthis prevents the flow of prana along with sushi humna nadi and inhibits the flow in our chakras and of kundalini shakti.

Brahma granthi is the first knot and is linked to mooladhara and swadhistana chakra. These are connected to our survival instinct and desires. When you get past the brahma granthi, kundalini energy gets an opportunity to wander up and

past the mooladhara and swadhistana chakra
without being drawn back by the instinctive
traits of our personality.

The second knot is vishnu granthi. It is linked
to manipura and anahata chakra. These two
chakras are connected to our emotional and
mental sides. Manipura chakra controls our
energy body (pranamaya kosha), and affects
digestion and metabolism. Anahata controls our
mental body (manomaya kosha). Together the
two together affect our physical body – annamaya kosha. To transcend vishnu granthi is to
no longer be bound to physical, mental and emotional desires. Relationships and energies take
on a different character and meaning and are no
longer limited to one's own desires and needs.

The last knot is rudra granthi, which is linked to
vishuddhi and ajna chakra. Vishuddhi and ajna
control our body of intuition (vijnamaya kosha).
When you get past the rudra granthi, identifying
with the ego stops. The experience of unmanifested consciousness appears in the ajna and
sahasrara chakras.

"Do not search, do not seek, do not strike, do not demand - relax.

If you relax, it will come, if you relax, you are there.

If you relax, you start vibrating with it."

SHATKARMA

In the old Upanishads you can read about Hatha yoga and how it is built up of shatkarmas, purification techniques. Shat means sex and karma – action. Shatkarmas consist of six different purification techniques. The purpose of Hatha yoga and shatkarmas is to create a balance between ida and pingala nadi, our two most important prana in the body, and thus also a balance and purity both physically and mentally.

Shatkarmas are also used to balance the three doshas: vata, pitta and kapha. According to both Hatha yoga and Ayurveda, an imbalance in the doshas causes illness. The techniques are also used before pranayamas and other more advanced yoga techniques to cleanse the body of toxins and to promote a safe and successful development purely spiritually.

Do not attempt to learn the techniques from a book. Seek instructions from a competent teacher who has adequate experience in the field.

Shatkarma include the following techniques:

1. NETI

A process where you clean the nasal passages. The techniques are called jala neti and sutra neti.

2. DHAUTI

A series of purification techniques that are divided into three main groups: assume dhauti (internal purification), sirshadhauti (purification of the head), and hrid dhauti (purification of the neck). These techniques cleanse the entire nutrient tract from the mouth to the rectum. There are four different techniques: shankhaprakshalana and laghooshankhaprakshalana which cleanse the intestines, agnisar kriya which activates the digestive fire, kunjal where one cleanses the abdomen with the help of water, and vatsara dhauti where one cleanses the intestines with air.

3. NAULI

A method to massage and strengthen the abdominal muscles.

4. BASTI

Techniques to clean the colon.

5. KAPALBHATI

Breathing technique to clean the frontal part of
the brain.

6. TRATAKA

A technique to develop the power of concentration by intensively focusing on a point or an
object. According to many Tantric yogis it is
the most powerful method of obtaining siddhis
(paranormal abilities).

The six shatkarmas consist of different varia-
tions of exercises. Advice and contraindications
should be adhered to. During pregnancy, only
jala neti (nasal rinsing) and trataka are recommended. While shatkarmas are cleansing and
invigorating, they are not the main purpose of
the techniques. Shatkarmas are done to promote the health of those who practice yoga, and to
awaken and direct the energies in the body and
mind safely so they do not flow the wrong way.
People suffering from any medical illness should
consult a competent teacher before doing any of
the exercises.

JALA NETI/NOSE RINSE

Jala neti is a purification technique that all yogis

practice before each yoga session. Jala neti cleanses the nasal passages and sinuses from mucus and contaminants. The air can then flow freely without obstruction through the nose. It counteracts illnesses of the respiratory tract and promotes healthy ears, eyes and throat. Tensions in the face are released. It has a calming effect on the brain. Anxiety, anger and depression are relieved. Jala neti stimulates nerve endings in the nose and promotes the sense of smell. A balance is created between the right and left nostrils as well as the right and left side of the brain. This, in turn, creates a balance and harmony between the body and the mind. The most important thing is that jala neti helps awaken ajna chakra.

"Who am I?

Am I my body, or can I experience it?

Am I my thoughts, or do I hear
them?

Am I my feelings, or do I feel them?

Am I my intuition, or do I sense it?

Who am I, I cannot be two?

I am the being, the consciousness,
the one who experiences everything.
In myself but also around.

I'm that, it's me. Om Tat Tvasi."